THE NEW NORMALITY OCTOBER 2020 EXISTS?

IT IS AN ILLUSION?

Same, better or worse

Fill in this space with your own handwriting:

IS THERE A NEW REALITY?

Reflect for you:

____

____

____

____

____

____

____

____

____

____

____

____

____

____.

THE NEW NORMALITY

OCTOBER 2020

¿EXIST?

¿IT IS AN ILLUSION?

Same, better or worse

By
DIEGO MARIN CHARRIS.,MD

Free Kindle Store Bestseller Author,
A BOOK FOR ME, IMAGINATION,
REALLY, WONDERFUL JOY,
APPRECIATION.

I dedicate this book
Being universal that I believe
To my mom, Electa
To my brother, Gonzalo
To Felipe
To the wonderful beings that
surround me
Thank you so much

CONTENT

Fill in this space with your own handwriting:

AM I PART OF THIS NEW NORMALITY?

____

____

____

____

____

____

____

____

____

____

______________________________________.

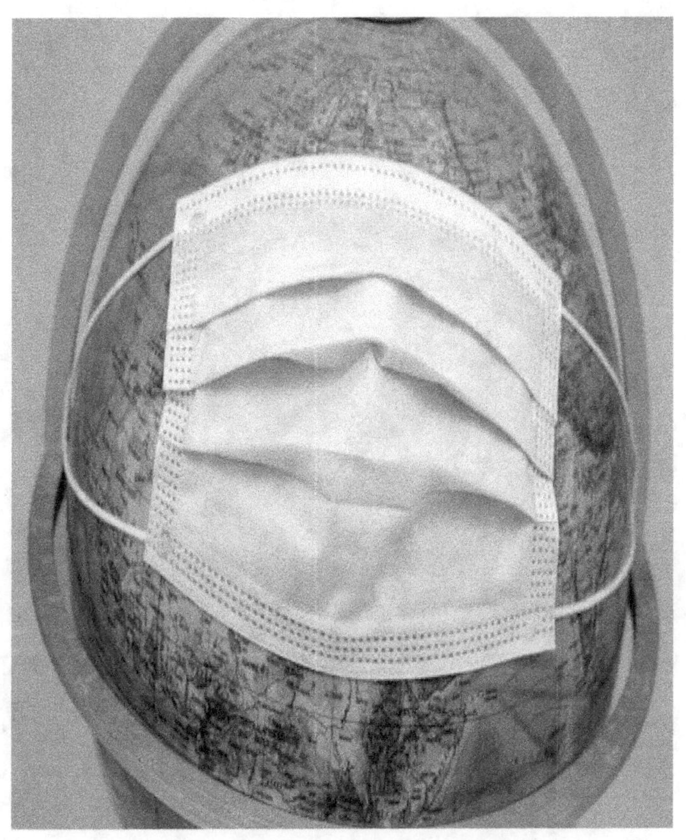

Image of Frauke Riether in Pixabay

INTRODUCTION

This is my very particular vision of the issue of normality since this October 2020.

You must have your own way of looking, of observing the phenomenon, you must exercise your capacities of attention, will, intelligence, to let your being flow and obtain the best life scenario that can be considered from consciousness.

I love to appreciate how inspiring our mind can be, committed to our survival, for what it is interested in, that we have given shape and attention to, it is fierce like a dog to its bone, but if it is not of its concern it fully contradicts itself, without judgments or morality.

Curiously, it speaks to us, it expresses itself, like that inner voice clearly saying that there is a duality, but that it is going to take the known path, we listen to it and let it work, in the belief that the known is always the best alternative in life.

On these bases we believe with blind faith to adapt to the events that modify the equilibrium state of our life, however, my own experience shows me that, we follow the same path learned from unconsciousness, although self-deception is the source of the incoherence that we live.

Overcoming an unusual event would be the example, we believe knowing is always to learn, however, the message is not learned, it does not overcome the barrier of unconsciousness, the typical model of incoherence that I have just pointed out.

Surviving witnesses of the 1972 Andes plane crash declared in their lectures that life after the event introduced them to the same routine that they estimated would be different after said tragedy, to reach the best level of being.

Starting from these premises, you know it, you see it, I see it, I know it, and yet it appears so imperceptible to natural sensors, and to states of being, that it is not appreciated from human consciousness, in an apparent and total denial of life, of illusion, of existence. Therefore, do we not see it? I ask.

The situation cannot be named, labeled, and therefore, it becomes invisible to the human species.

In the state of nature a phenomenon is transformed in the same way, as I have described it, with an evident intangibility, I mean the development and growth of each individual of the species from birth to death.

In other words, during each moment we are physically changing and we do not perceive it, in spite of it it is happening.

In a similar sense, the natural environment varies, the movement of the earth, the solar flow, the climate, are different in each season and we do not appreciate it although it overwhelms us; Even the infrastructure of cities is not the same as our childhood, and yet its appreciation goes unnoticed from the conscious point of view.

Each environment described and not perceived is producing a direct or indirect effect on the existence o

The species is facing the same experience at this time.

The changes have invaded the system little by little, entering the gravitational field of life with the aforementioned effects, and we have not seen it.

First television, then the incipient computers, joined the Internet chain in the 60s, in the following decade mobile phones, with their intelligent prospecting, social networks and technological platforms increased the penetration of homes, jobs, leisure and fun, modifying current patterns of mind and action in a continuous, constant way.

And this active dynamic has crossed the field of humanity's existence throughout fifty years, within the framework, even of a new century, and despite its great impact and adaptation, it has not been perceived under a high standard of consciousness. .

I mean, in our hands wanders an arsenal of impressive technology (intelligent mobile - it surpasses us), loaded with applications, advanced software (although we are its source, we marvel), which have modified human practices, redirected by those media without appreciate it in its reach from the global mass of beings.

We are satisfied with its use, but not with its effect disguised as a benefit, despite the justifications.

These stealthy changes have come to invade the scenario of money and its dematerialization, the digital, cryptocurrencies are a reality, plastic money the second invasion, then financial applications for the management of banking products, and the reduction of working capital in cash; only numbers circulate the technology networks creating a different panorama of uncertainty for each generation.

Fearful older adults when going to these media, alarmed by the absence of evidence of their wealth and assets, made up of numbers in accounts that they only see when they withdraw cash from an ATM.

Those of the transition see the two worlds in appearance, the old one of the security of their parents, and the new one of the digital age with its benefits in the process of its induction.

And finally the new generation, children of the 21st century, who already belong to the contemporary industry, willing to live in and out of technology, now from their homes in daily life and work added, with entertainment from the small television, mobile phone or super-smart, with transactions with its cellular cards, dynamic keys, plastics, and belief in a sophisticated standard of transactions of this level, perfectly adapted without contradictory existential flows now.

So, we contemplate with admiration, this event is becoming apparent right now, in front of us and we do not notice it.

The change accelerated dramatically in a short period of time, the catalyst was a global situation known to all, expected and unexpected, a multitude of films from the last century on television and in cinema warned of the phenomenon, the history of humanity narrates similar events.

The man in his high power of appreciation, in spheres of control and dominance, observed human behavior, that is, they noticed the limited observation capacity from the consciousness of men, the foolproof survival factor, and the option to change as an imperceptible variable, and they decided to use it to order the world in their vision.

The planet in the last century was upset in all its evolution, the habitat was contaminated to the point of the commitment of life for the advancement and industrialized development.

The population and favorable living conditions expanded the number of beings, conventional activities were saturated, the physical spaces of work and housing stopped satisfying the demand, the monetary system to the point of collapse, with two substitute crises, social movements began to organize, violence increased in all its forms, money in its ordinary transaction models was not enough; the investment and performance processes did not allow the desired returns; the great capitals reduced in its expansion with limited markets and full of new immaterial ideas in all countries to bear fruit with dynamics and "human work".

This apparent chaos deserved urgent measures and renewal, when the variables of change had already been introduced at the end of the 20th century (multifamily, large marketing areas and coexistence shopping centers, social networks, international awards, computers, terabytes, information superhighways, for example), without the expected result, due to the resistance of the generations in transit, a population that took a long time to welcome them as culture and wrap them up in everyday life (home automation and immotics).

And now the ground has become fertile to achieve those tasks of economic and social reorganization at the level of the entire human planisphere.

The motivated emotions and the low vibration increased due to fear and the lack of certainty, the success of the new measures, in force, to modify habits, trends, uses, customs, forms, norms, fashions, etc.

The phenomenon causes my curiosity, and I am going to study it in the next chapters, well, it seems novel in all its aspects, but deep down it is appreciated that technology is the only noticeable change, but the uses are the same, money is the Source of the model, although today it is digital and immaterial, markets are nourished by the same exchange of goods and services, and evolutionary human nature, not in its model of biology, but in its identity, personality, and interaction without variation, the same beings Middle Ages with similar responses to the typhus pandemic of the Middle Ages survive today into 2020, you would believe.

Therefore the initial premise of this writing finds foundation in the arguments of the introduction, we know it, we perceive it, we notice it, we see it, but we do not appreciate it or make it conscious for the life of each individual, the global mass is dragged in numbers without form or content, simple statistics without any added value, therefore, analysis is relevant for self-recognition, self-inquiry, reprogramming, on the way to regain happiness; Integrated mind and consciousness found the tools to resume existence from its foundations, which are not precisely technological.

A close friend heard my speech on one occasion, and objected with a statement, he predicted, - it would not be possible for you to spread your literary production of vital reflection in a massive way, without the current state of the art in the media and specialized platforms, sentenced.

To which I sincerely replied, -Your precision is true, but you forget the fundamental thing, this wonderful task would not be necessary, since human beings would live happily in their daily lives migrating like nomads in all the lands, habitats and natural environments of the earth. , enraptured by their environment and the inspiring scenes that would accompany them from their birth to their transcendence into another being. He was silent.

IS IT REAL OR ILLUSION?

The bias of the mind can induce confusion that we understand or comprehend as realities without being it.

It has been well said that contemporary man lives from his mind, and creates the realities that his material of memories and experiences condenses into a source of assortment for thoughts and imagination, and there a natural error of conceptions and visions of the world that surrounds him.

To minimize this option, it would be convenient to outline which situations are the ones that trigger my observation of the current state of the planet, to specify, and reveal if this flaw is documented in this text, or if on the contrary, it is not a mental illusion, and it is a reality that the senses can capture, although at the level of unconsciousness, for now.

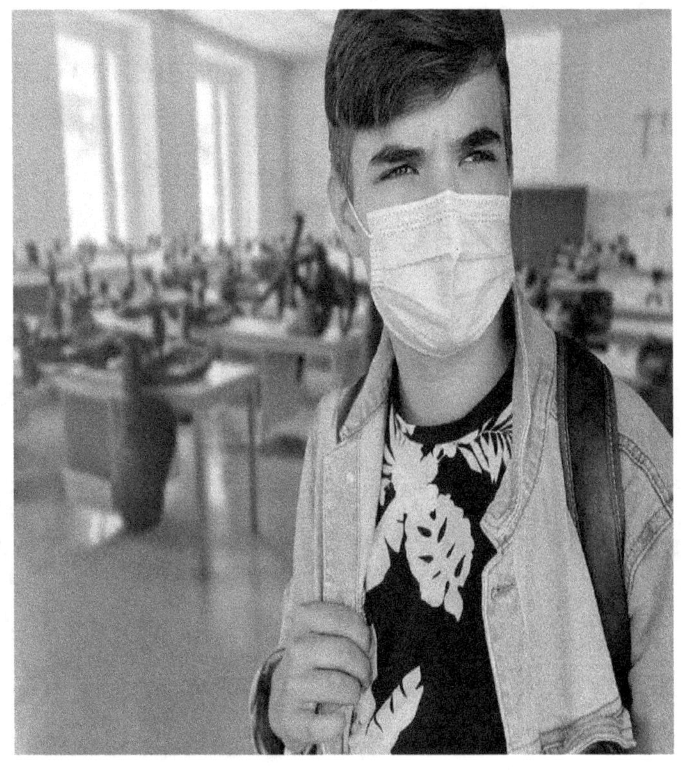

Image of Alexandra_Koch in Pixabay

BEFORE

So, before the worldwide spread of contagion, from a source in the Chinese community, the planet, as we have already hinted, was quite convulsed by particular situations that threatened world stability, some of which were a reflection of the dilemma:

1.   The fall of traditional authoritarian systems such as Gaddafi in Libya and Mubarak in Egypt redefined global politics since 2011.

2. The capitalist economic model, and the democratic system in decline.

3. The trade war between China, Europe, the United States was in the news in that period before the virus; the dollar was devalued, the yen and the euro were strengthening; Yuan at values of the 2008 crisis. Depreciation of emerging currencies; indebtedness at intolerable levels of world economies, even the American debt exceeded reasonable limits. Russia and other states in a plan to recover their currencies, massively bought gold, today they sell it.

The US gold reserves do not cover current cash or obligations to its creditors.

Insolvency of European economies such as Greece, Spain and Turkey.

4. Unemployment, work stoppage, of the predominantly young active population spread like the pandemic, the G8 countries affected in a similar way to the United States.

5. Conflicts between Iran, USA; USA, Russia; USA, Korea; The world and Venezuela, oil in the middle.

6. "SARS and MERS outbreaks controlled."

7. Protests and indefinite global revolutionary movements, led by youth and university students, seeking labor, economic, climatic, social, educational demands: Yellow vests in France, Indefinite strikes in Spain, France, Brazil, Germany, Chile, Colombia, Bolivia, Argentina, Peru.

8. The world climate in chaos due to generalized industrial and vehicular environmental pollution, global warming, storms, floods, tsunamis, yellow and red alerts in large cities that do not give in to restriction measures affecting the health of citizens.

8. Massive migrations of Africans to Europe, refugees die every day in the process. Rejection of these economies to the human crisis. Venezuelans migrate to neighboring countries due to political crisis.

10. Teleworking was a global normative reality, but it had not been possible to encourage the planet's population to massify it, appreciate its advantages and disadvantages, employers did not take leadership and actions in that

sense due to distrust of the operators.

11. The orange economy had been established on world agendas, hand in hand with teleworking from home, or active private rental spaces (cooworkers), actions in addition to well-regulated entrepreneurship, and entrepreneurship, but not very effective in their impact on the market. labor.

Situations as a whole that required immediate attention, to reduce the consequences; States and the staff of young leaders in a generational change of technocrats in the presidencies and heads of government demonstrated the inability to efficiently resolve situations.

And by chance of fate, the COVID contagion wave appears, which triggers a contest of situations that numbs the minds of the world population for a prolonged period of at least six months, possibly more.

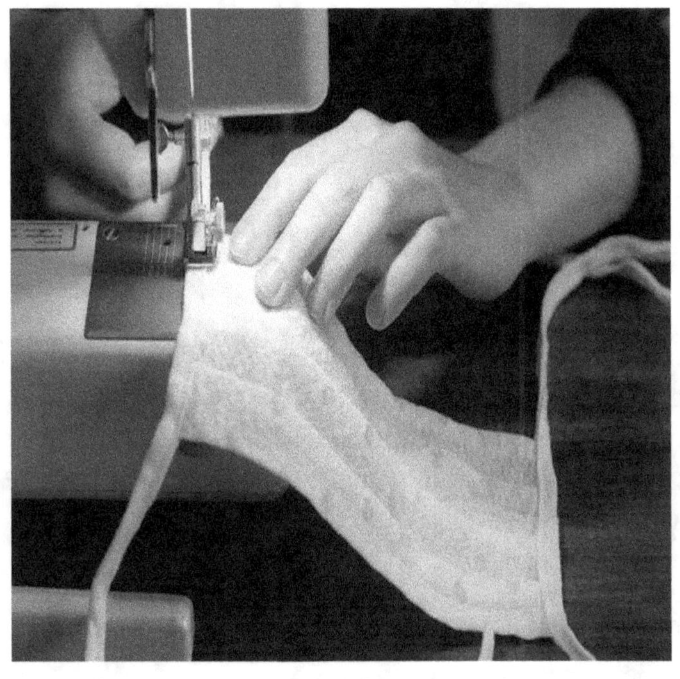

Image of ivabalk in Pixabay

DURING

Period that allows me to make the following additional observations:

- *A great coherence and consonance of world leaders at all levels of government in the face of the viral global dilemma, in terms of actions, policies, periods, quarantine, restoration of normality, actions of staying at home, closing of shows, measures of prevention, vaccines, work from home, maintenance of food supply, imports of basic products, border closures, reduction of internal mobilization, migration, etc.*

- *In the same way to go out to the "new normal."*

- *Integration in particular in the group of OECD countries, faced with a random and untimely situation, a somewhat strange phenomenon given the differences that are usually observed between these leaders.*

- *The isolation measures affected the domestic economy of the population and the businesses, and although measures were taken to alleviate them insufficiently, they generated the closure of many businesses, problems with leases, and debt of the population, returning control to the financial markets crowded with debtors, product of grace periods, and relative relief, increasing the interest charges and the amount of the installments at the end of these relative and ineffective means of help.*

- *Communication systems terrorized citizens, encouraged the information of fear and pandemic, creating high levels of uncertainty in citizens, using statistics that are difficult to verify, and information from medical care centers, where despite exposure. Fortunately, professional personnel suffered the least, however, from direct exposure to the biological contaminant.*

o *In an unusual way in the mass media, especially on television in the midst of the pandemic, the offer of commercials was unlimited, all in their content adapted to the situation, in total congruence with the policy of care, isolation, Home delivery of products without contact, a suggestive situation, since the advertising and marketing agencies, models, and their staff were locked in their homes like any citizen since the beginning of the massive contagion.*

- *In the opposite direction, but with the same efficiency, now in the new normal, the message of self-care and staying at home disappears, and the supply of products to the home is restored with greater intensity using technology and applications.*

- *The same situation was experienced in local supermarkets and department stores; In the week when the isolation periods began, these establishments were full of all the products and lines, an incomprehensible phenomenon since the employees and food factories were in the same isolation situation, despite this they continued to operate as the same way even with more momentum, despite the risk reported in the media and governments.*

- *The common global denominator was the capacity of government systems and measures, even at a coercive regulatory level, to isolate the population in their homes regardless of their health, economic, labor and social status.*

- *During the period, there was common agreement that the vulnerable population was that of the elderly and the elderly, since the studies do not specify which ones, indicated that contagion was a risk for this population, young people and children did not belong to this niche Was the virus selective about its preferences?*

- *The dynamics of trade increased throughout the world through digital platforms, APPs, computers, electronic commerce, bank transfers, payment through dataphones, without physical contact, even days without VAT were released to mobilize businesses, with great reception by the cloistered population.*

- *The hospital and ICU systems collapsed due to patient numbers; The health market increased in this particular area, with massive purchases of ventilators, diagnostic tests, and the establishment of additional structures for benefits in extra-institutional environments, now there is a massive and global business with the subject of vaccines.*

- *Isolation made it possible to free the environment of the cities from vehicular pollution, with a significant reduction in the figures, the other species relaxed a little from the polluted life of man.*

- *In the same way, space was used to improve the locative infrastructure of roads and roads.*

- *Local and world television opted to repeat old programs, novels, repeated films, remakes, violence, affective dramas, taking advantage of the confinement, they united old and new generations using content proven for its effectiveness to establish parameters of behavior in the population.*

- *Isolation increased levels of family conflict.*

- *Similarly, it demonstrated the addiction of all generations to digital information from computers, social platforms and networks, cell phones, and applications; human interaction followed this line of predominant behavior in youth.*

- *Education demonstrated that the model perfectly adapts to any system, as long as enrollment is canceled and that happened, the communication technology through the internet supplied the processes without defect, few universities or colleges delayed their programs; Teachers and students massively communicated through this means, evidencing the insufficiency of the evaluation systems, and privileging the content and information to create value in the process. The educational infrastructure was not relevant to the system.*

- *Formal state jobs stood out for remaining in their actions, communicating with the community through digital means without obstruction of global dynamics, even taxes and tributes were canceled in a timely manner, most of them virtually as much in person.*

- *The private sector found evidence of the lack of need to lock its workforce in offices, performance from home even for large call centers developed smoothly from home, despite the fact that many of them handled confidential data information from Your clients.*

- *The church and its rites became widespread, the message spread through the networks and television without an obstacle to its end, virtual donations replaced face-to-face donations, the communities understood the preeminence of the indulgence model through the virtual payment of bank transfers.*

- *The holy father demonstrated his faith and belief by modulating the communiqués and faith on a universal level in the same massive systems.*

- *The global discussion on the true origin or not of the pandemic was the subject of discussion in all kinds of media, with dissimilar positions, without certainty of the definition of the subject.*

- *The rate of common violence, of guerrilla movements, and the independence conflict, of traffic accidents, and common and work-related diseases of diverse origin was reduced.*

* *Global events, awards, concerts, sports activities could be held without human presence, with indicators of success in virtual assistance.*

* *Telework, telemedicine, orange economy in networks worked and were accepted by the citizens of the planet, and employers as a valid offer for the performance of individuals and organizations.*

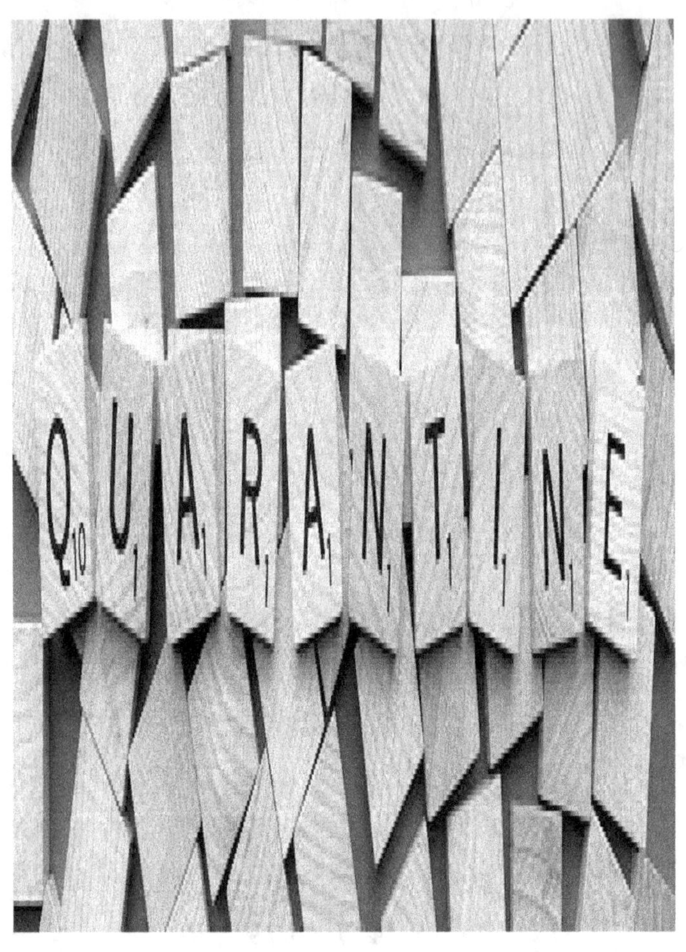

Image of Wokandapix in Pixabay

THEN

In this stage of "**new normality**", particular dynamics under study are appreciated due to their effect in the medium or long term, **which tend to restore the usual state of things,** a somewhat different before, based on the human being's ability to forget, Finding yourself living from the unconscious mind, and surviving "adapted" to your current programming with minor lifestyle modifications.

I mean, the movements of the human mass adjust at this moment, to the same phenomenon that happens when a norm changes a situation of any kind, the initial response a complaint, then some degree of express manifestation and revolt, then a period of acceptance and finally the norm is fully established and nobody rejects it, it is fulfilled.

Exemplary of the case, led to the integration into the life of the large urban communities of the so-called **peak and vehicle plate**, restricting mobility, to reduce environmental pollution, without affecting the payment of high taxes, or restricting the production of vehicles, or its sale.

In this temporal space, other observations arise for your reflection, dear reader:

1. The government systems have overcome to some extent the state of discomfort of the population in sensitive issues, visible in the past, even strengthened in their power of

coercion, assuming more radical positions in other senses, now without opposition due to the persistence of current and subsequent biological hazards.

2. The issue of vaccines, the new waves of contamination that youth with a better immune response have begun to suffer, and even children, have allowed the relaxation of the isolation and confinement system, without the use of special medical care units before the satisfactory recovery of young people exposed to this virus, with mortality rates maintained in the elderly population, as has been prevented by the system.

3. The full reestablishment of the tabloid and alarmist news on television newscasts and in other

media, once again encouraging violence of war, common, transnational, then political, then economic and finally social, abandoning the radical interest of the virus and the "pandemic", with some isolated notes, and the use for now of virtual means to integrate the commentators and experts from their homes.

4. Mass advertising on television for health and disease products was fully restored; exponentially the economic sector pounced on the population loaded with consumer messages, for now towards virtuality, digital consumption from homes.

5. The working model of basic productive sectors with the presence of employees is almost

completely normalized, despite the persistence of the risk of viral contamination, without an increase in the relative numbers of patients, and without vaccines.

6. The official sector provides its services in a mixed way with a level of efficiency higher than the traditional face-to-face from virtuality.

7. The private sector of goods and services works in a mixed face-to-face and virtual model, resuming its levels prior to the peak of pandemic and confinement.

8. The health sector remains stable, therefore, its performance was ideal and constant during the viral crisis, small adjustments in terms of prevention and contagion have

been added to its healthcare provision actions.

10. The vehicular flow increased to usual levels, the contamination returned to its path, the restriction similar plans to those prior to the pandemic.

11. General sectors such as hotels, tourism, bars, restaurants already show recovery figures and begin to care without fear and relaxation of isolation and protection measures.

12. The banking business came out stronger, its business figures increased, the use of platforms showed its usefulness in transactions, the webs were modernized, the service assistance processes were improved due to the reduction in the flow of customers to offices, customer

service virtual from home of officials and employees effective.

13. The public transportation system is beginning to reach its traditional congestion levels despite self-care measures. Air travel tends to normal at the national and international level without a substantial increase in the pandemic, "the virus is controlling itself."

14. Sightseeing has been restored with the summer vacation period around the globe.

15. The population confined to homes is more adapted to the circumstance, they perform fewer actions on the street, they are

more specific in their movements due to the apparent risk.

16. Citizen protests have subsided, some peaks isolated by violence from police officers, and their abuse; rebellion against the mask in Germany; political movements on the issue of elections reappear with force, etc.

17. Sports, churches, and shows in large crowds are waiting for their own space, as the pilot exercises are not showing greater risks for the population with masks and minimal spaces of separation between individuals.

18. The tendency to return to the face-to-face model is more active every day in schools and universities.

19. Food production on the planet was not affected by the pandemic, nor was the handling of industrial processes for its transformation.

20. Cross-border trade was never affected in the pandemic, nor was the transport of food or its storage, activities that have remained constant in variation.

22. Technology demonstrated its ability to keep human beings locked up by carrying out work, leisure, entertainment, leisure, business, and service actions without any defect.

23. The global figures for mortality in the pandemic, in a strict sense, did not exceed the current population averages by countries and common causes throughout the

period of confinement and new normality.

24. Human beings in the world were confined for several months and survived the experience of being locked in their ordinary means of life; poverty, wealth, debt, family conflicts, illness, emotional dilemmas, and emotional states were maintained. Common and armed violence decreased notably.

25. The cost of food and basic consumer products increased substantially due to necessity.

26. An evident generational change was revealed, a predominance of youth over adulthood, in all areas of life, an uncomfortable phenomenon for the species, when it has not evolved in terms of

inclusion and equality, and education facilitates discrimination .

Surely I miss many aspects that you have considered my friend.

The obvious question and others after these simple and surely few observations before, during and after, would be:

What happened in these months?

The example of the story of the lying shepherd boy takes effect, the wolf comes, the wolf comes and ever came.

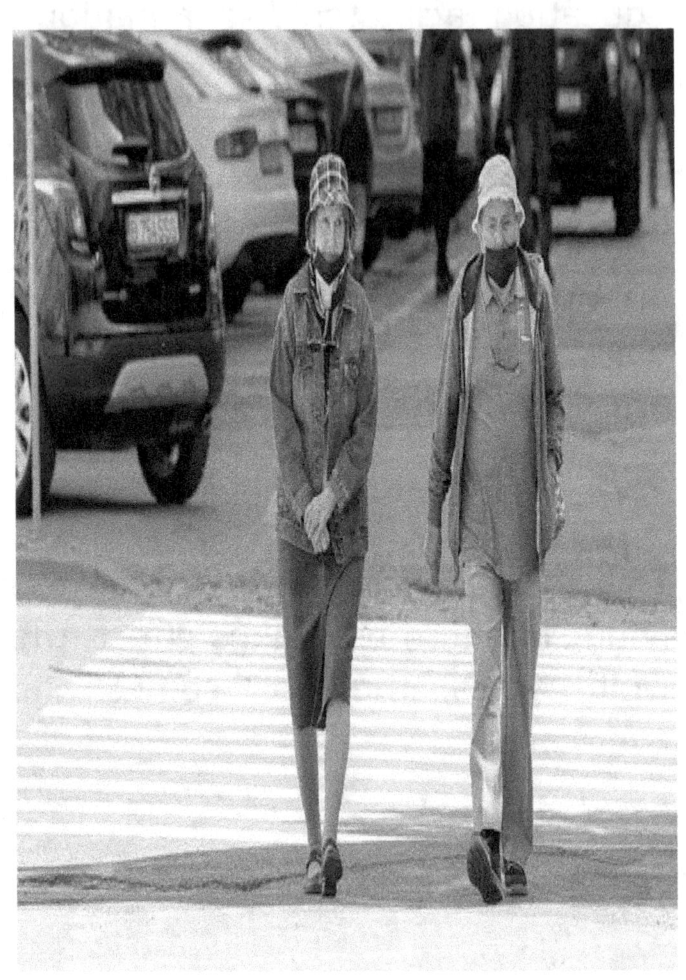

Image of Candid_Shots in Pixabay

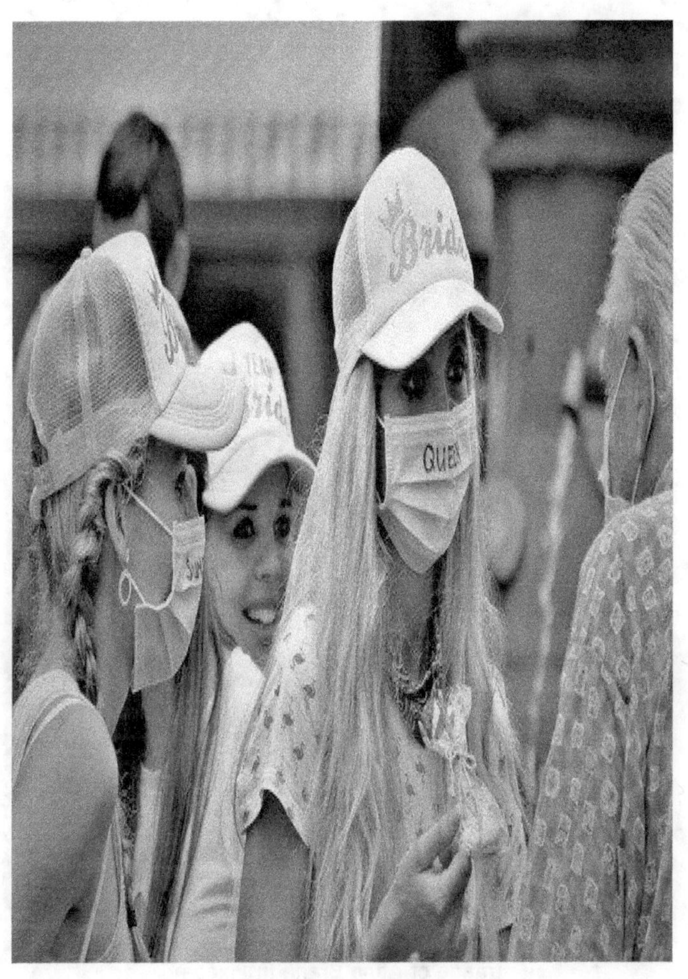

Image of pasja1000 in Pixabay

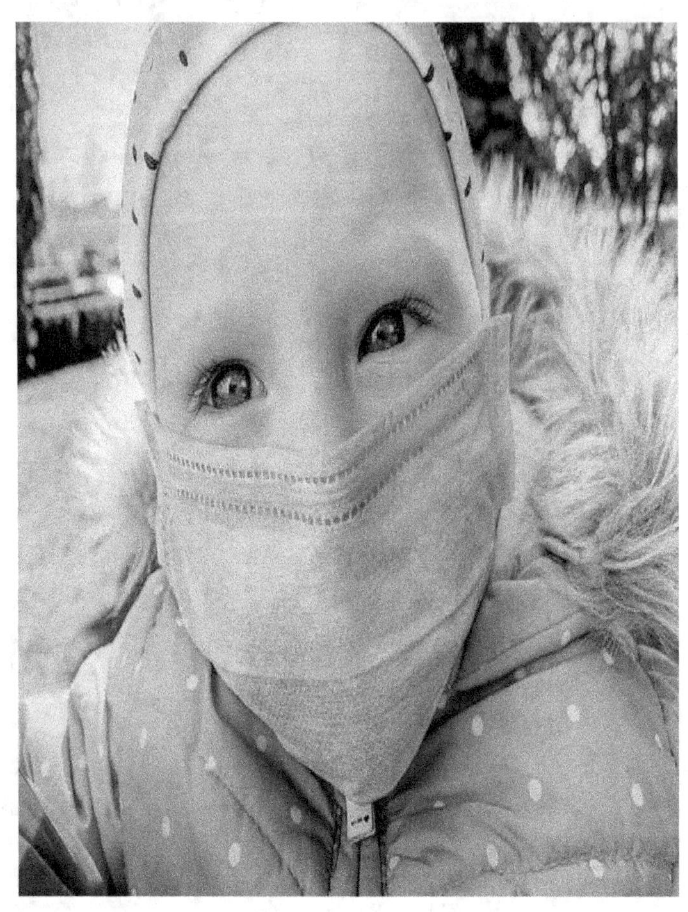

Image of Alina Braha in Pixabay

NOW

Let us mention some trends to continue moving forward without judgment, about what could change something before humanity, which now appears again as before but now.

- Some multinationals have decided after this experience of confinement and work from home, a definitive model of mixed work, home for several days and in person at the company according to need, prioritizing productivity and results over the place of performance, under a different leadership style.

Siemens and Twitter highlight the news taking advantage of technology, they are at the forefront of the cost reduction model, and increased benefits for their employees. Facebook Inc. and Alphabet Inc. have made it easy for their operators to work from home for the remainder of this 2020 season.

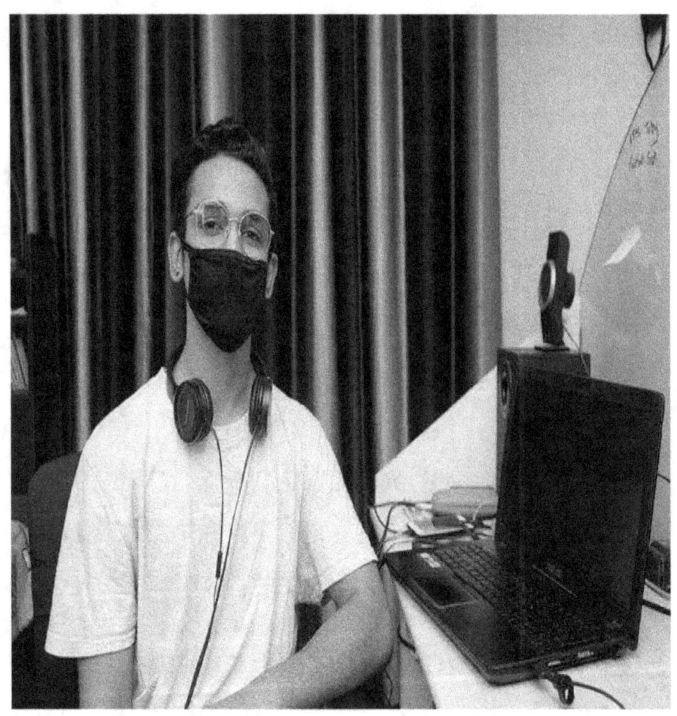

Image of Yogendra Singh in Pixabay

- Studies have been prepared that justify the cost management of organizations from the public and private, to develop work from home in a definitive way (remote work or from home) of their employees, who apparently have become accustomed to this reality .

- Both employees and employers have found performance levels in home work that are up to thirty percent higher than in-person work.

- The current dilemmas of contact between office workers for care have disappeared in this period; personal friction does not occur for obvious reasons; bank tellers are more relaxed due to the substantial decrease in the public they serve; in the same way, officials of receipt of documents, invoices, and attention to the general public perform better from virtuality, receiving electronic documents, emails and answering in the same way.

- Laws that seek to facilitate this type of remote work are passed in the legislatures of several countries, for example, subsidy for homework equipment, respect for active working hours, tax deductions, compensation, more lax hours, etc.

-On the table of discussions of experts and scientists around the world, topics such as: the global prevention of new episodes such as the current one; the change of the capitalist model in its organizational structure; the needs of the species over the economy, prioritizing well-being over business income; Different management models, and encouragement to shareholders against performance per se; The purpose as a measure of efficiency and organizational performance is current academic debate oriented to solutions for communities not only for the increase of profits without measure.

-	The education system demonstrated its weaknesses for students of all levels, particularly the university, who appreciated:

- That more can be learned from home, with fewer distractions and social and academic stress.

- It was evidenced that the academy is a social environment rather than training, and that dilemma is resolved in favor of learning as a useful life purpose.

- In the same way, it was observed by the human conglomerate that the costs of the academy are exaggerated by the mere fact of attending some facilities.

- The physical displacements to the study site have been shown to translate into unnecessary substantial living and economic costs for the student and their domestic economy.

- In the same way, the little need to migrate to other cities to acquire remote knowledge was identified; academic entities in any contemporary location can attend training sessions all over the planet thanks to virtuality.

- It was highlighted that social networks integrate youth under a notorious range of normality, and that social integration spaces are not limited to the study site as a definitive socialization advantage.

- At the level of secondary education, the habits of human relationship between parents and children improved, with greater integration even from the academic point of view, sharing work and education, recognizing added value to mutual help.

- Teen pregnancy and sexually transmitted disease rates fell in those niches.

- University students, especially from the areas of engineering and administrative training, highlighted that face-to-face workshops and academic mural and extramural practices can be significantly reduced without affecting performance, since the theoretical stage is always higher than the effective one in laboratories.

- Students observed that urban planning can be improved and large academic spaces can become living, relaxation, and distraction areas for exercise and other tasks.

- Academic administrative processes are facilitated through electronic means.

- The level of food and nutrition improved in the students during this period, due to the elimination of junk food from their diets, in addition to the significant savings in money for this unnecessary consumption.

- The closing of the schools once again demonstrated the

value of training from home with principles and values from home taught by parents and close relatives.

- Through virtual education, schoolchildren strengthened new attention and cognitive skills and abilities.

- The teaching staff was the most affected as they managed to cover a greater number of students with few teachers. The recording of the contents and the preparation of the materials increased and improved the level of training of teachers from home, and of students alike.

- Absenteeism was significantly reduced due to the concern of parents directly immersed in the processes, motivating young people and schoolchildren to their daily tasks.

- The common illnesses resulting from the contact of young people in their academic environments decreased significantly as shown by the global figures.

- The habits of boredom and initial discomfort of the pandemic were modified, to more relaxation and happiness in students at all levels.

- An important number of basic level students, significant in the population with the lowest economic resources from the public sphere, was affected by the absence of computer systems in their homes to receive remote training; in addition to the increase in the domestic economy in public service expenses, unsubsidized food as happens at school, malnutrition, family violence; detecting the communities that the satisfactor is dependent on the State in these cases of notorious inequality.

- Many of these positive effects of the academy are extrapolated to work environments due to their obvious benefit, in terms of cost reduction, efficient cost management, increased affectivity, better emotionality, fewer vital risks, increased productivity and performance, Health & Wellness.

- The so-called pandemic, released a situation that was not appreciated for some years, the option of repopulating geographic areas affected by the viral situation; Several cities, communities, and regions of the world offered migrants economic incentives, and incremental living conditions of comfort and well-being, for minimum periods, particularly in technical areas, for young couples to live in these neighborhoods.

- The proposals of multilateral organizations for the prevention of epidemics are active, in this now.

- Global health models, organizations at the same level, national and local, demonstrated their strengths and weaknesses, processes that are beginning to bear fruit in terms of valuable information to improve and provide feedback in all areas of the global health systems. Circumstance highly dependent on the economic development of the states and their government policies on the matter.

- The pandemic impacted life habitat to some extent, particularly in vehicle pollution, carbon emissions, and energy demand management; In spite of which the climatic changes and disaster advanced throughout this period with devastating effects, great forest fires, plagues, cyclones, clear waves, floods, typhoons, alluviums.

- The contraction of the economy and unemployment is evident worldwide; factors such as tourism and remittances have been strongly affected; the balance of payments of some countries require credit support in an altered global economy; the course of economies is unpredictable under the gaze of committed leaders under the gaze of multinationals that neglect local needs.

- The infrastructure of the cities showed weaknesses that facilitate the spread of diseases, the way in which businesses, public services, multifamily, organizations, industries, healthcare systems have been conceived must be reassessed.

This is a very incipient panorama of my global observations on the dynamics of the pandemic in its different edges and moments, therefore it has the bias of my partial observation, which induces me to take sides, and declare that the world phenomenon at the beginning is both reality as an illusion from the most important perspective, the human, for that I proceed to resolve the doubt that I raised a few paragraphs ago that happened.

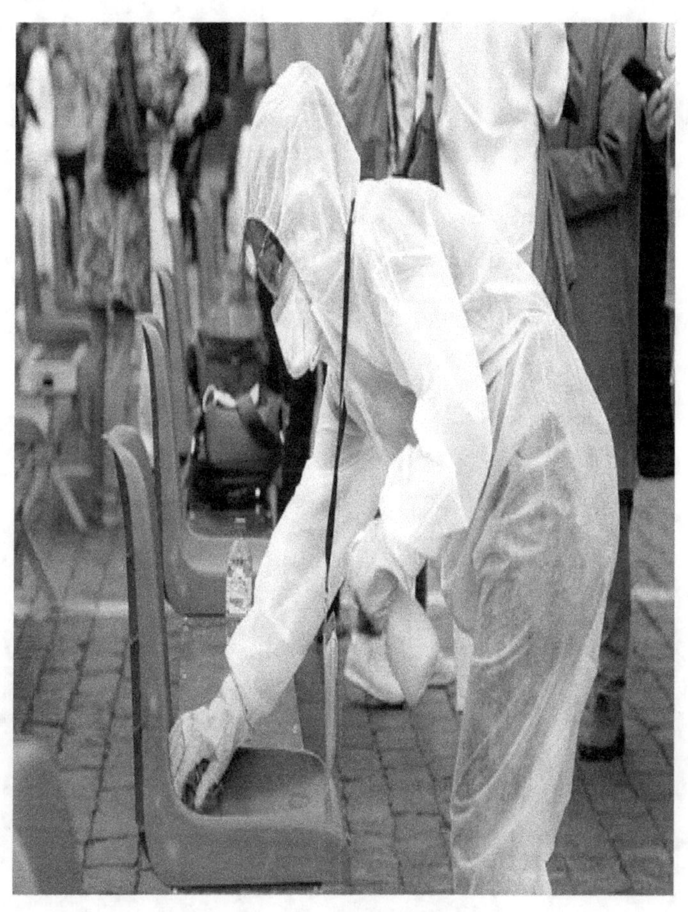

Image of klimkin in Pixabay

WHAT HAPPENED IN THESE MONTHS?

It is a complex matter, since we are immersed in the living space of presumptions, assumptions, and these are necessarily the product of prior information and memories, of the logical analysis of evidence from the past, and therefore useless, if you can exceed the parameter please use it.

A reasonable questioning arises that directs my understanding to define the basic question formulated, Did production or innovation predominate throughout these months? We are going to determine it.

The only change that dominated this period was a fact that was consolidated since the first wave of humanity, when primitive man gave value to fire, now it is called cutting-edge technology, artificial intelligence, nanotechnology; and we only reduce ourselves as a population and mass to the screens, without going into the knowledge of the technology that creates them, and less of their contents that direct the existence of humanity.

My natural sense tells me that human life in this century therefore revolves around screens, television, computers, cell phones, movies, drones, video games, which are concentrated through the content created by various sources, without our consent, the life that we must follow, despite each individual having free thought, autonomy, free will, conscience and will.

Then, the screens reflected and reflect the content that has generated this situation, transmitting updated news from the world, reporting a situation in China, which the WHO later determined was global in scope, and after the global and national decisions that led the population to confinement.

The decisions of local governments communicated through these means induced unusual behaviors in that isolation, determining that life would develop predominantly from home, as a protective measure for the prevention of massive contagion in the community.

Thus, life followed its usual course with restrictions, suggesting that humanity was at risk and that is why the way to protect the most underprivileged was in that way, as indicated by experts and the scientific community, without other alternatives, so as the subject would have been approached in the Middle Ages.

The ignorance of the species, and the power of the rules, supported by the authorities, in addition to the vision of the media, made that reality visible without prior consultations to make consensual decisions, a general circumstance throughout the planet.

The mind of the species created the illusion and the phenomenon came to life in each individual from their own perspective, assuming a passive role, for the survival and conservation of the vital state due to the risk perceived from unconsciousness.

Associated variables such as domestic economy, previous health status, finances, housing, services, food, work, associated activities, were unknown and the cave, the confinement was the basic and primitive measure of protection in appearance, the consequences were not They mattered, governments ordered, and intimidated citizens as individuals and families kept the order without analysis.

The situation was presented as untimely, sudden, random and high risk, unexpected.

Space was freed for food, markets were crowded and the subsistence economy of higher price and consumption was structured for several months, the media created the illusion, the figures highlighted the evolution of a global pandemic that was trying to be controlled by the prevention of contagion be to be.

Hence, illusion dominated reality, the unconscious mind over the conscious.

Production determined the course of life, and in that scenario family activities, education, and work were immersed, using the screens again, while other economic sectors were reactivated (# quédateencasa), however debt collection persisted and relief was heavily touted in the medium term.

Thus a dynamic of life and work was established that demonstrated or at least simulated a new lifestyle.

Space used for social proof that could not be applied in any other way: For example using technology from home for work; the performance of social platforms throughout humanity for the integration of the species; the use of financial means through APPs and massive plastic money; the provision of services from technology to the home; the invasion of programming content through the media in a massive way; the decontamination of environmental pollution created by industry and motor vehicles; the avoidance of movements, revolts, strikes and social protests; changes in the structure of the social model, remote work, generalized remote study; integration of the family with the return of the woman full time to the house; the identification of vulnerable human groups through voluntary enrollment in state programs; discriminated censuses; identification of tastes, preferences of individuals and nuclei; performance of companies in providing services to the home as in the 60s and 70s; measurement of the reduction of common, armed violence; and accident rate, among others.

We continue in production dominating innovation in this endemic process, this only becomes transparent in the development of ventilators for respiratory assistance, and in research neglecting protocols for the

development of vaccines against the virus.

Unfortunately this valuable space of human experience induced by unknown things, circumstances or people, has been completely wasted by governments, individuals and social nuclei, we are returning to the before in a very advanced way, and quickly.

In other words, we return to daily life with a mask, to do the same as always, the exercise that has intensified the most is the provision of services and work remotely, that is, from home, and the attention of needs from home by companies to the same destination using technology and telephone platforms.

Something similar to the decade of the seventies of the last century, where milk was delivered to homes, laundry was delivered at home, women were engineers and housewives, and residential areas were the preferred places for companies to door-to-door sales.

Little did the dilemma of man, of the species, of unconsciousness, dehumanization, corruption of the soul, human interaction diminish inequality, the purpose of life, respect for the other, dignity, delivery to spirituality, love as a divine mandate, wisdom and integration with nature.

On the contrary, the isolation was total, the beings looked at each other with distrust, with fear, the buildings of horizontal property seemed prisons where no one could relate to anyone; fear displaced medical personnel due to its high degree of contamination and transmission; human contact was isolated, motels were vacated and the clandestine kingdom all over the planet of those confident in their pleasures and the absence of fear of a news to which they gave little credibility.

A simple exercise of existence under these real needs unleashed him when he requested financial help from different individuals in the world, from close friends to millionaires recognized in the networks of the planet, and a response of community unity was presented: It is a difficult situation, I do not have money, I live on my salary and it is not enough, we receive many requests for donations, if I could with great pleasure.

None of these beings was congruent with the moment, their minds, despite the apparent risk, told them that they were going to survive for a long time and they required resources to maintain their status forever, immortal men living a pandemic of mortality, I would say.

What has happened then?

Our most intimate desires have been manifested, and no one can deny it, the sun has shone without clouds.

Initially we have believed the information, and that has been facilitated by the fact that within us exists as such that incoherence with the universe, that opposite sense is full of abundance, prosperity and happiness, in addition to everything for everyone, without exception, now and in everything instant.

That is why we accept I include remote work without hesitation as a reality within the illusion, well, we want from unconsciousness to work that way, free of supervisors, discomfort with co-workers, traffic, offering our best work version without the need for sanctions , mistreatment, contemptuous looks, etc .; and this space is created by desire, and the universe delivers it fully.

We are consistent, we appreciate rest and leisure time, and we know that by working efficiently from home we can have a better standard of living by working, it is a human desire and the pandemic attracted it as a life option in total congruence.

For this reason, students and parents, concerned and in search of ways out of their economies to educate their children, have attracted knowledge of reality, and have massively recognized the phenomenon.

The universe has revealed in the pandemic, and the father son binomial has realized that university tuitions are very expensive due to the fact of providing hotels and face-to-face actions, our being understood a contradictory message and aligned with the universe, That is why in this period he showed us that there is a need to change the model, which all humanity now sees.

For example, an intelligent young man pointed out to me that there is no longer a need to attend face-to-face conferences with international guests in each profession to appreciate their perspectives from another continent, you only have to go to the internet, communicate with that expert, offer him the money he considers worth. the fair service for its training, and make it visible to a whole country of students through the systemic medium that we most want, virtual video platforms, postcast, television, and others.

In the same way, we wished not to have to travel from our city of origin and learn in recognized universities and that reality that was tangible for postgraduates now took on relevance for undergraduates, colleges, schools.

The abundance becomes clearer in this pandemic scenario, given the coherence of beings, of students, inasmuch as the universities have a large amount of recorded class material, which facilitates the repetition of the subjects at any time, without the need for additional notes, students can consult them as many times as they wish, and the cost of universities is substantially reduced, professors can remotely build their chairs with much more care and abundance.

The grandparents taught their grandchildren the existence of basic classes for schoolchildren through television, it was called educational television and they longed to return to the same, because, that reality within the illusion is beginning to come to life by desire and the universe It condenses it, for the classes with fewer resources, the television is always available, only a public policy is required, and employment is created, the education message is disseminated, and it is validated with the experience of many years ago effective.

In the same way, the pandemic returns the desire that the house, the home be the source of wealth for society and families, and in the less well-off strata, this desire was longed for, and therefore, the option arises of taking schoolchildren to their homes door to door snacks from public services, breakfasts and lunch so that children maintain their adequate nutritional status, instead of moving them to schools, as a means to avoid massive infections, and their infrastructure, devote yourself to other better actions.

The pandemic has demonstrated the effectiveness of the home marketing system, this avoids unnecessary travel in vehicles, the congestion of supermarkets, and squares, now with a call, or a video call, we can bring the supermarket back to the house, to residence, saving substantially money and time, these hypermarkets can be eliminated by bringing products from source to consumer creating a network of valuable production and innovation at factory prices.

The neighborhood store model is based on the same system, they have long supplied households with their addresses, and agents by bicycle as the network businesses.

The monies from large surfaces can perfectly continue to mediate if it is their wish without the presence that has proven to be a source of disease and discomfort for humanity, creating vehicular chaos and pollution due to the accompaniment of travel always in public or private motor vehicles .

Walking has become a routine of life, which favors health and well-being.

The illusion of the pandemic has created the possibility of modeling and using the best, changing the before for an innovation before, however fear paralyzed the population and few developments were made by the government, individuals and organizations to move radically towards an incredible world.

Only, restraint and isolation models, face masks, plastic visors, disposable gloves, separators between public service conductors and their customers, and synthetic meshes were created to isolate one employee from another in work occupations, medical tests and vaccines in development.

The long-term vision was not appreciated in world leaderships, that is why the same news, the same shows, the programmed mind of each other is only restricted to what he knows and knows, football, tennis, musical shows and cinema, no we advance in understanding the planet and its liberating message, when we have the powerful tool of desire, and the universal unity that gives us everything without limitations.

We have limited minds, due to unconsciousness, but we can get out of that confinement, humanity asks for it, it is the integration of being with other beings overcoming the scarcity of the life system, it is a proposal of the universe that has been reflected from the mind of many individuals who reflected on this period and it takes universal force.

What do we do? Is the basic question now.

I repeat an example, which demonstrates the power of the coherence of thoughts and the universe, if I want to kiss a beautiful woman I know, I will always reach that phenomenal moment, it is possible because I want it from unconsciousness and from consciousness, in total coherence and congruence, the universe, and the activating reticular system, the brain amygdala lead me to fulfill that desire always.

In the same way, I do believe and let myself be influenced by the negativity of the media, of advertising, messages penetrate through my senses and that is the illusion, the unreality, the lie that induces me to attract what I do not want to. the powerful and divine existence that endows us in joy and abundance.

The opposite route is available all the time for our well-being, that internal struggle that bothers us is the desire to join the creative universe to get out of the confinement of the mind and enter a new dimension, that of certainty, that of truth, that of unity, that of love, unconditional, that of prosperity in the material and spiritual without diseases, without pain, without suffering, all in a state of universal wealth, this is a clear message of this period that now, they want to start cover with the model from before.

WHAT DO WE DO?

The new normal is an illusion, it is a programming message from the outside to the inside, as has always happened.

Let us note that if the life we witness today does not make us happy, it is the product of our thoughts, the emotions and feelings that derive from them, that is why it is possible that the universal complaint has manifested itself in this way, because happiness and joy does not reign on earth in this age.

WHAT DO WE DO? We simply must regain the power of the inner being, and attract what we want, understand it as already granted, and project it on the screen of our life and the universe.

What does that mean for programmed and practical minds?

It is a simple task, in the beginning you do not have to do anything.

Observing what we think is the source of change because we make conscious what works unconsciously.

And then seek coherence of desires and thoughts without denials, allowing, eliminating resistance, and accepting that we cannot control anything, the full path for the message of abundance of the universe to penetrate.

In other words, dissipating dualities, wanting and not wanting, loving and not loving, having and not having, believing and not believing.

This coherence eliminates the fear and contradiction that fracture the message of well-being; If you do not know and do not know what the universe attracts for you product of your most intimate desire, ask it with love:

- **Creative Universe teach me what you have granted me, that I do not see, and I deserve.**

And this message, how is this practice digested in this situation?

Simpler still.

Do not resist, say thank you, and watch the universe act, just focus your attention on what you want, my book "My wishes knew it", guides you.

Let's see how it works from my perspective, yours will always be more valuable because it implies that you have expanded.

So:

If you have been working remotely from your home for several months, and they offer you to do it permanently, and you liked how you have performed, now for taste and preference, accept.

Even the call centers of the large companies in the sector have observed the advantages of having their employees working at home.

If you have been aware of the process, make a list of the advantages that you have had and enhance them, do not evaluate the disadvantages.

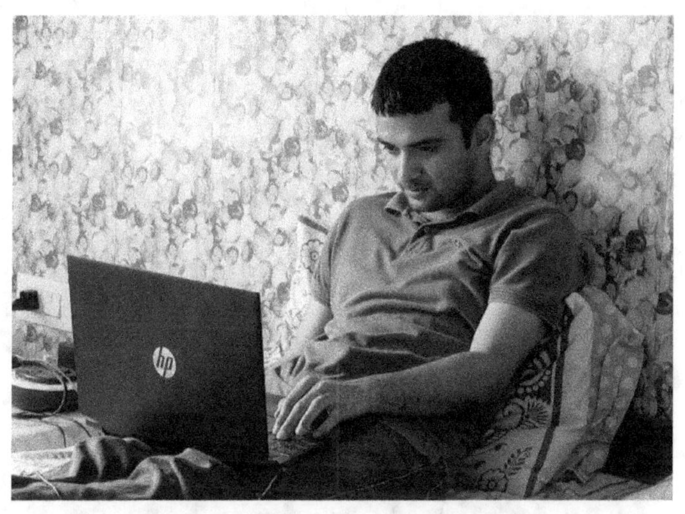

Image of Rajesh Balouria in Pixabay

For example, the comfort of working from home, the options for rest during the day, the possibility of walking and exercising, sharing meals with your family, saving on travel by vehicle or public service, reducing risks contagion, freedom from the control of bosses and middle managers; the ability to complete your tasks more efficiently and effectively, self-recognition, and self-inquiry, etc.

If you don't like the path traced and you want to stay in the programming model, resume your conventional work with prevention measures.

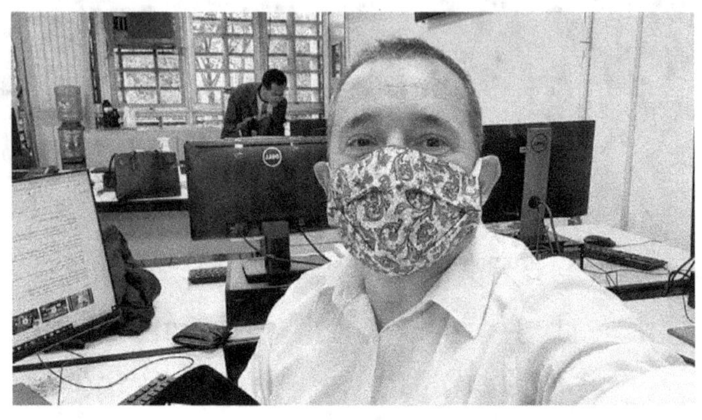

Image of Luciano Teixeira in Pixabay

You have survived the impact of the system, you can now select your suppliers at home more specifically, by quality, costs, service, offers, discounts, and if you want to go to a supermarket select the one that suits you; walk, visit parks, play, and if your family has joined the remote model from the education and work of your loved ones, well, enjoy.

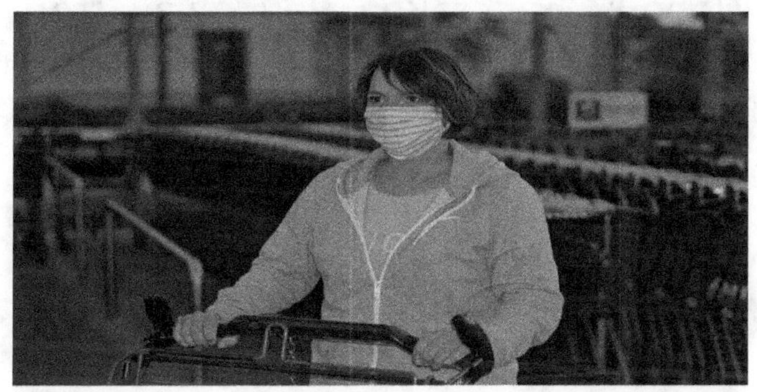

Image of Anrita1705 in Pixabay

Select the internet service networks according to your business project, check the domestic economy, plan the television programming you want.

Check the study model of your children, and if the remote offer at home continues, it privileges the advantages in terms of finances, schedules, availability, network, quality, safety, teenage pregnancy was substantially reduced in this period for example.

Nobody has taken you away from your friends, family and neighbors, if you suffer a change, it is your mind that does not settle, reviews the thoughts and enters into coherence, you can visit them, find yourself in public spaces, take a walk, taking certain care, go ahead.

I am optimistic, the changes are for the better, however, I foresee that this period will not last long, the benefits for human beings will soon be detected by the system and we will return to the same as before.

While this phenomenon lasts, channel your energy in your favor, it is your best ally and that of your family.

Observe, this period allowed you to discover that you are not work, you are not a student, you are not a compulsive consumer, you are not a tourist, you are not your family, you are not what the outside wants you to be; You had the opportunity if you saw it, to find a valuable being for yourself.

In this sense, you were able to heal, recover your self-esteem, your emotional relationship, your eating habits, walking, distraction, leisure, well-being.

How do we do it? letting the inner energy flow, and watching us, our universe expands, and at the beginning we see ourselves very small, because, we were dominated by the system, worries, work duty, the selection of the place to have lunch, the digestion in the middle of the day of work, exchange with many beings in public spaces, loneliness in the midst of people, addictions to pollution, cigarettes, drinks on weekends, all situations that have been overcome thanks to doing and changing for this period of lifetime.

Despite the evaluation I am doing, I know first-hand that your mind is only focusing on the main tether of the mental system: Money, and debts, and managing that reality, illusion.

This topic from the most advanced version of being, in the dimension of the universe, is resolved, it is so abundant in our lives, but we do not give it space, precisely because of those thoughts.

I mean, if I think I need money, I am lacking; since I always have the abundance that I require of everything in this life, the creative universe provides, if I project the lack, well, the message of prosperity does not arrive and I stay with the projection of lack, it seems quite absurd but it is.

In any case, if you think you can be in control, assume your power, responsibility and create new sources of income, based on your skills, knowledge, and penetrate the system from home, for consumers from home for now, if you return to the routine of Face-to-face employment, it will be easy to adjust to the life you led, you just have to deny the benefits of this wonderful period.

Few beings on the planet have recognized the advantage of this situation, multifamily families can integrate a whole network of services and functions, alternating activities, with great financial savings of unnecessary costs and expenses, but it requires respect for others, admiration and understanding of human nature.

Purchases adjusted to economies of scale, especially for products and consumer goods, food, hygiene, medicine, snacks, taking advantage of the fact that large companies are willing to take home orders. In a similar order, the use of shared vehicles to travel in different activities; or the rental of services for this option saves fuel, automotive wear, and pollution, as an example of adaptation to normality.

With a greater sense of belonging to the species, from the home, shared economic funds can be managed to minimize the impact of indebtedness with the financial system, with greater privileges between neighbors, or professional services with greater rationalization of fees.

Education does show a notorious impact, because of the evidence that I reveal in this space of global human existence, the opportunity to force a change is in our hands to significantly reduce the effect on household finances.

Few professions, technical or technological actions, secondary and school education cannot be taught and learned remotely, significantly reducing costs of tuition, travel, food, housing, clothing, health-life risks; increasing comfort, resourcefulness, and life stocks.

Audio and video webinars are the powerful tool of virtuality today for education now; Teachers at all levels must adapt to this context, since they are a minority facing the dense population mass dedicated to studying.

It is that studying is a pleasure in life, not a business, its strength consists in inducing satisfaction for personal development, therefore, the pandemic created this possibility, we must leave the minds programmed to forget the diplomas and certificates and mutate them into conscience and service.

This leaving the walls of colleges and universities carries an important added value, the socialization imparted outside these training centers is much more liberating, special, friendly, consistent with beings, with life, with expansion. The academic stronghold generates a confusion that has led to the current pathological state of life in the communities, due to the competition that is hostilely integrated into education originated in labels and stereotypes, which discriminate against an individual throughout their life (Nerds , geeks, bullying, etc.)

As the development of the situation can be seen, the most notorious and dark, due to its radicalization, is related to the immateriality of money, nor will cryptocurrencies be necessary, the currency is disappearing as required by the system, the bills are expensive, its guarantee in gold impossible to maintain for central banks, therefore, everything will be reflected in numbers in cell phone accounts, encrypted cards in mobile phones, and in QR codes, Bar code, with sensors in all businesses on the planet, such as China and Japan have been carrying out for a decade, in their street advertising, and supermarkets, taking the products home at the preset hours, here we do not have any action for our benefit.

Image of Tumisu in Pixabay

In appearance, so for now there has been a change, I would believe the appreciation is not true, the system had already been modifying reality (illusion) for a long time so that you would not notice it, this period was the final phase of this first stage of programming for the planet's species.

To cook frog legs, they are introduced into warm water and little by little the temperature is increased until they are cooked and they do not even notice.

Your responsibility in this process is to be happy, and if you understand it quickly, you will be more so.

You already knew about the advances of digital technology and the exchange through cell phones; you already knew about network marketing; You already knew about cookies and the pixelation of your tastes and preferences from your emails, from your visits to social platforms; You already knew about mass entertainment and advertising on networks; you already knew the tabloid handling of television and the violence of programming; you already knew about the orange economy; teleworking, entrepreneurship from home; of the PPPs and their banking model; You already knew about the integration of countries like the OECD, and those of the East; You already knew about the change of models in China from low-quality producers to cutting-edge innovators; You knew about the economic dilemmas of the USA, Europe, Latin America; From the media, cinema, television and multilateral organizations that the pandemics were close (outbreaks of SARS, cholera, malaria, dengue, chikungunya, Ebola in Africa).

As you can see, you are simply not aware of your environment, only of what the media presents you in their news and how the orientation changes every day you forget, but not your powerful mind that stores the information, you are surprised by the panorama, but now Did you know.

In the same way, you let daily life manage your routine, and you do not see any further, work, money, accounts, concerns of the family environment, work, fear, routine.

How we do?

Stop, stop, sit down, rest, the world and life continue to evolve, contemplate, do not identify yourself, accept your identity in unity, occupy yourself with it from consciousness.

What do you appreciate?

Nothing, or everything, there is a new normal, better, worse or the same.

That perception does not matter for the universe, it is programmed, your past is being expressed, your memories.

Feel, the sensations reveal to you if there are tangible changes, if the moment makes you happy, cheerful, you smile, and yours at home express themselves in the same way, there is a change for your well-being, if nothing happens, your feeling is flat , you find yourself caught up in the dynamics of the world as it was before and as it continues to be.

If you complain and you are a victim of the situation, you are not happy and you are in frank involution, stop the step, stay still, and allow the universe to take control, and expand you.

Changing for change is the mentality, adapting is a valuable

tool, always with a predominance of the inner being.

This event has not occurred from my criteria in this short space of universal movement, the dominated species accepted the illusion without response on the planet, without its consent, accepting without controversy, as happens daily, a system that obscures existence, its expansion, the freedom, love, therefore we live from the mind, requesting indulgences and confused.

The circumstance is dependent on the fear of transcending, which in the East for millennia was part of education from childhood, or in Greece was taught to youth, today it is denied in the Eastern and Western world, and that fear induces the responses of the humanity that have been integrated along that path into the so-called Pandemic.

A situation common to life, was expressed in an alarmist and careless way, instilling panic in humanity, and believing to subject beings to their domination and change in response to social dilemmas, they have favored to some extent the expansion of their lives, I hope that those who made it persist on that path, happier, more joyful, more enthusiastic, more inspiring, more fulfilling, more enjoyable.

EPILOGUE

After this brief process of understanding some situations derived from the global episode generated by the governments of the world and the media, **I find that normality is just another label,** the profound changes announced are few, but if we take advantage of them in our favor, they are forceful.

I have tried to discover some topics, surely you, dear friend, will broaden the perspectives.

This human condition becomes an opportunity to regain the **"normality of being"** by definitively leaving the mental programs and living in pure consciousness.

The obstacle to the life of well-being is **fear,** and its unfortunate interpretation associated with it with death and money.

Overcoming these barriers of being is possible, it is required to look inward, deeply, and stop controlling, letting go of the human experience, and living only as other species do.

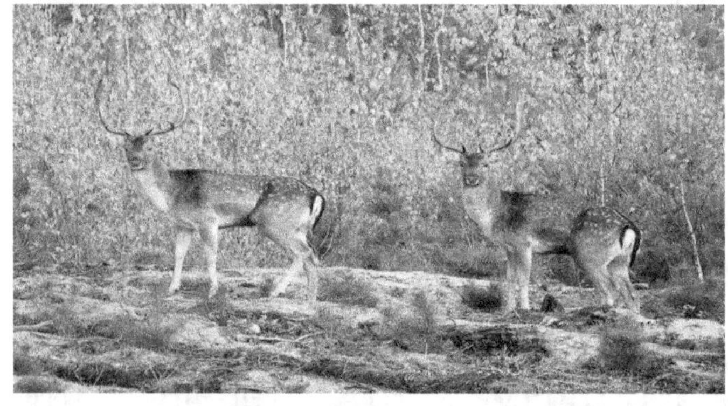

Image of Krzysztof Niewolny in Pixabay

The identity of each one of us as the source of real change persists, then advance in the consciousness of self-recognition and end the path with the understanding of the existence of a universe that offers us everything, satisfying the most intimate desires, if we accept that we cannot control anything and we surrender to that wise and superior force.

I have offered a number of strategies to address this illusion, which exists as reality in the mind, but not in the world created by the universe, they are simply induced expectations, which have been labeled as a **"new normal"**, the same as always, that of before, but now temporally and geographically, not at all a real component of being, therefore, it is not a reality, it is an illusion and only you are responsible for leaving there to recognize the fullness and well-

being of existence now, in the
presence.

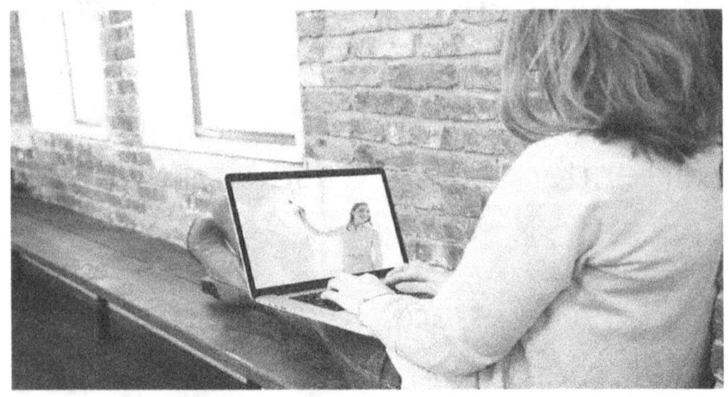

Image of mohamed Hassan in Pixabay

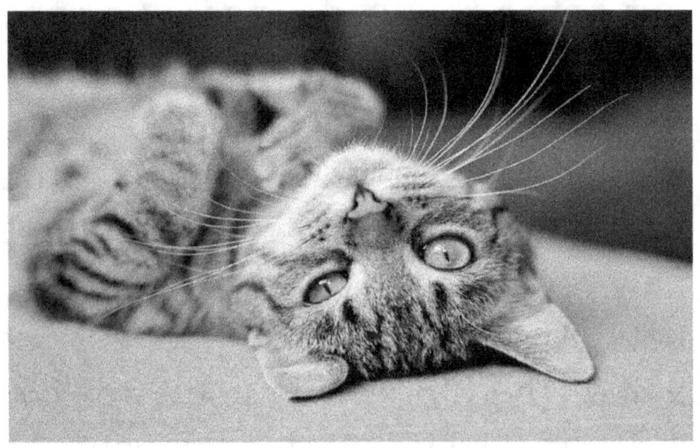

Image of Daga_Roszkowska in Pixabay

I agree that the "new normal" is regulated?

I believe The "new normal" is a
matter of economics and finance?

Education in the "new normal" should be?

Are we human beings moving towards consciousness in this pandemic?

Do I understand self-care in the
"new normal"?

The pandemic for me was?

Do I think about remote work?

GOOD LUCK

THANKS VERY MUCH